Feline Fine!

Homemade Cat Food & Treat Recipes –
A Cool for Cats Cookbook

BY

Daniel Humphreys

License Notes

Table of Contents

Introduction

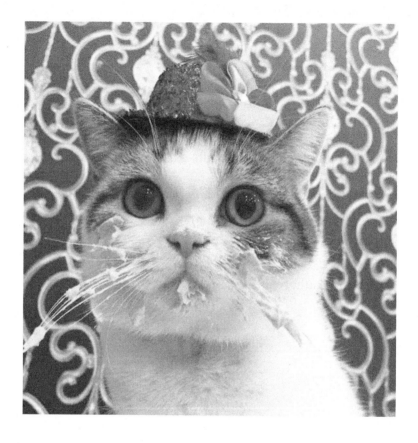

While lots of dogs can easily digest a number of different foods cats need to eat meat, and avoid indigestible carbohydrates. In fact, they need double the amount of protein to dogs.

So, cooking for cats is the perfect way to ensure that your feline friend is getting the amount of nutrients they need.

Once you have decided to prepare you own homemade cat food, it's advisable to talk to your veterinarian in case he, or she has any advice or suggestions.

Once you are happy, very gradually switch your cat over from store bought food to homemade. You can do this by introducing one homemade meal each day over a period of 7-10 days.

Remember too, that treats and biscuits should never exceed more than 10% of your cat's daily calorie intake. Also, just because your cat loves tuna, salmon and cheese it's advisable to feed these in moderation only.

Also take into account that kittens, senior cats, and pets suffering from allergies, food intolerances and health conditions will have different dietary requirements. Your vet will be able to advise you on which foods are not suitable for your cat.

Follow these homemade cat food recipes and you will have a purrfectly healthy cat!

A Cool for Cat's Cookbook expresses quantities in yield rather than servings. Portions depend very much on the size, weight, age, and fitness levels of your cat. Most of the recipes in this cookbook can be stored in the refrigerator or freezer.

Birthday Cake

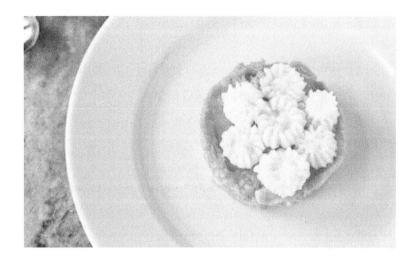

Cottage cheese is the best cheese to use as it is safe for your cat to eat.

Yield: 2 cakes

Total Time: 25mins

Ingredients:

- 1 (5 ounce) can tuna
- 3 tbsp. plain cottage cheese (mashed)
- 3 tbsp. coconut flour
- 1 medium egg (beaten)

Directions:

1. Preheat the main oven to 350 degrees.

2. In a mixing bowl, combine the tuna along with the mashed cottage cheese, coconut flour, and beaten egg.

3. Stir well until incorporated.

4. Pour the batter into 2 cups of a lightly greased muffin pan.

5. Bake for approximately 20 minutes.

6. Serve as a treat.

.

Boiled Chicken

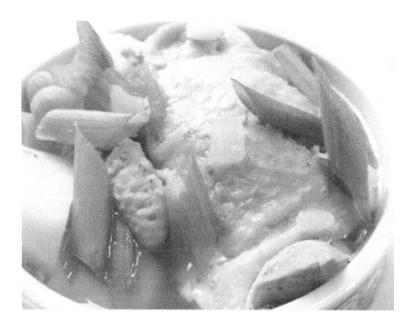

A healthy dinner for your feline friend thanks to the protein from the chicken and the high levels of fiber and antioxidants from the veggies.

Yield: 3 cups

Total Time: 5mins

Ingredients:

- 2 cups chicken (boiled, bone-free)
- ½ cup broccoli (steamed)
- ½ cup carrots (steamed)
- Chicken broth

Directions:

1. In a food blender, blitz all 4 ingredients until you achieve a cat food consistency. Add a drop more broth if you feel the mixture is too dry.

2. Allow the cat food to cool before serving.

3. You can store any leftovers in an airtight container for up to 7 days.

Catnip Soup

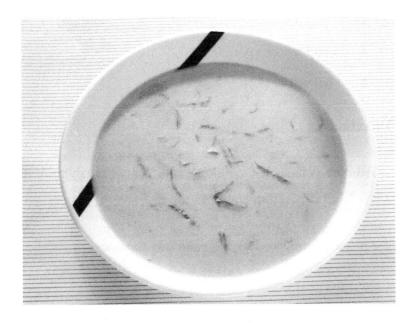

You can serve this soup either cold or warmed in the microwave.

Yield: 1

Total Time: 2mins

Ingredients:

- ½ cup dry vegan cat food
- ¼ cup warm soy milk
- 3 tsp catnip

Directions:

1. Add the vegan cat food along with the warm soy milk in a bowl and stir well to combine.

2. Sprinkle catnip over the top and mix together.

Cheesy Homemade Cat Treats

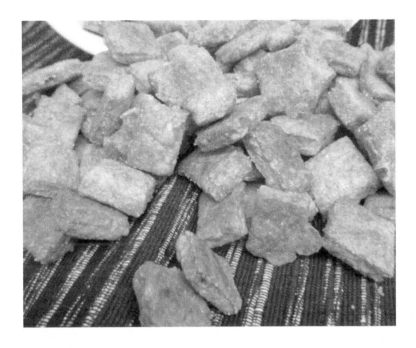

Homemade treats are economical and easy to make but remember cheese is a treat and must only be given to your cat in moderation.

Yield: 50-55

Total Time: 30mins

Ingredients:

- ¾ cup cheddar cheese (shredded)
- ⅓ cup Parmesan cheese (grated)
- ¼ cup plain yogurt
- ¾ cup white whole wheat flour
- ¼ cup cornmeal
- ¼ cup water

Directions:

1. Preheat the main oven to 350 degrees F.

2. In a mixing bowl combine the cheddar along with the Parmesan, and yogurt. Next, add the whole wheat flour and cornmeal.

3. Add sufficient water to the mixture to make a workable dough. Using your hands mold the dough into a ball and then roll out to a square of no more than ¼" thick.

4. Cut the dough into 1" sized pieces and arrange on a lightly greased cookie tray.

5. Bake in the oven for approximately 25 minutes.

Chick 'n Biscuits

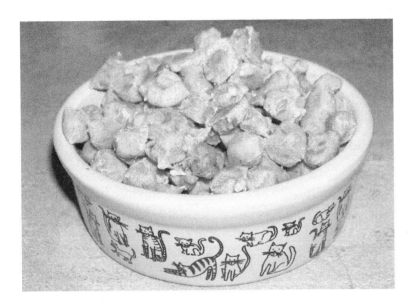

Tasty bites that will have your pet asking for more!

Yield: 18

Total Time: 30mins

Ingredients:

- 1½ cups cooked chicken (shredded, bone-free)
- ½ cup chicken broth
- 1 tbsp. soft margarine
- ⅓ cup cornmeal
- 1 cup whole wheat flour

Directions:

1. Preheat the main oven to 350 degrees F.

2. In a mixing bowl combine the shredded chicken along with the chicken broth, and margarine and blend.

3. Add the cornmeal and wheat flour and mix.

4. Using your hand knead the dough mixture into a ball and roll out to a rectangle of no more than ¼ "thick.

5. Cut into 1" sized bite-sized pieces and arrange on an ungreased cookie tray.

6. Transfer to the oven for 20 minutes.

Chicken and Pasta Dinner

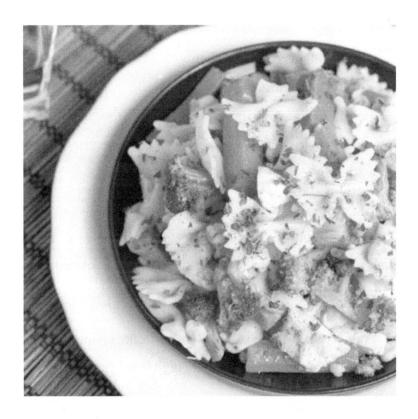

Pasta should only be given to your cat once in a while so if you occasionally have any leftover pasta; your cat can join enjoy a little along with some protein-rich chicken.

Yield: 2-3 servings

Total Time: 25mins

Ingredients:

- 2 tbsp. vegetable oil
- ½ pound ground chicken
- 1½ cups chicken stock
- 1 small carrot (finely chopped)
- ½ cup macaroni

Directions:

1. To a medium sized saucepan heat the vegetable oil. When hot, add the ground chicken to the pan and cook until the chicken is no longer pink.

2. Pour in the chicken stock, along with the chopped carrot and macaroni and over medium to high heat bring to the boil.

3. As soon as the mixture is rapidly boiling, reduce the heat and simmer for 12-15 minutes, or until the pasta is tender.

4. Remove the pan from the heat and allow the mixture to completely cool.

5. When the mixture is sufficiently cooled add it to a food blender and process until the ingredients are combined.

6. Transfer the mixture to an airtight, lidded container and store in the refrigerator for up to 72 hours.

Chicken and Rice

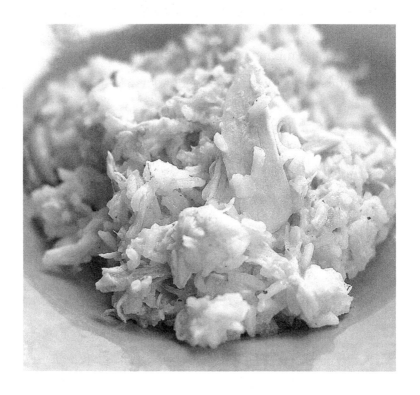

Plain food, including cooked chicken and boiled rice, can help to soothe kitty's GI system.

Yield: 2-3 servings

Total Time: 5mins

Ingredients:

- ⅓ pound boneless chicken breast (raw weight, cooked, chopped)
- 1 large egg (hardboiled, chopped)
- ½ ounce clams in juice (chopped)
- ⅓ cup long-grain rice (cooked)
- 4 tsp canola oil
- ⅛ tsp salt substitute (potassium chloride)
- 4 bone meal tablets (finely crushed)
- 1 multivitamin, mineral tablet (crushed fine)

Directions:

1. In a mixing bowl add all ingredients and stir to combine. Serve at once, refrigerate or warm a little before serving.

Chicken and Vegetable Stew

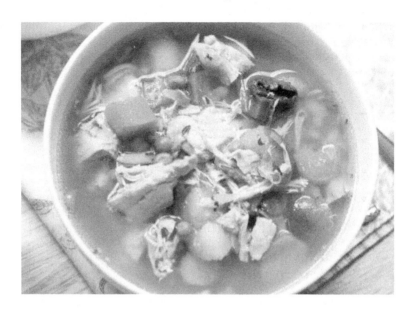

A tasty chicken and veggie stew that can be made and stored in the freezer.

Yield: 6-8 servings

Total Time: 45mins

Ingredients:

- 1 whole, free-range chicken (bone-free)
- Cold water
- 6 stalks celery
- 8 carrots (scrubbed, not peeled)

- 2 yellow squash
- 2 zucchinis
- 1 small broccoli crown
- Handful green beans
- 2 cups brown rice

Directions:

1. First, wash the chicken then place in a stew pot and cover with cold water.

2. Chop the vegetables and add them to the stew pot. Next, add the rice.

3. Cook in an oven set at 450 degrees F for 10-15 minutes. Reduce the temperature to 350 degrees F and roast for 20 mins per pound in weight, or until the meat comes away easily from the bone and vegetables are just tender.

4. Completely debone the cooked chicken. It is crucial that no bones remain as these are dangerous for your pets.

5. Transfer the stew to a food blender and process until the mixture is bite size and a coarse consistency.

6. Leftover stew can be stored in the freezer in Ziploc bags.

Chicken Ball Treats

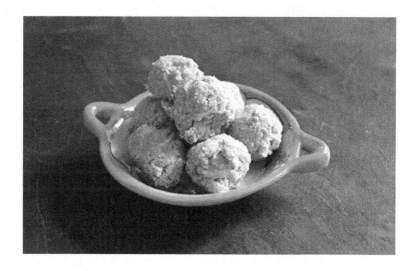

When doesn't kitty crave a little chicken now and again? This quick recipe will give your cat lots of chicken treats to enjoy.

Yield: 18 balls

Total Time: 30mins

Ingredients:

- Margarine
- ½ cup of whole-wheat flour
- ½ cup of powdered milk
- 1 cup pureed cooked chicken
- 1 tbsp. cod liver oil

- 1 large beaten egg
- ¼ cup of water

Directions:

1. Lightly grease a cookie tray with margarine.

2. In a mixing bowl, combine the wheat flour along with the powdered milk.

3. In a second bowl, add the chicken along with the cod liver oil, and beaten egg. Mash the mixture until combined.

4. Add the chicken mixture to the dry ingredients, gradually adding water until a sticky dough ball forms.

5. Using a scoop, form small balls and arrange them on a cookie sheet, approximately 1" apart.

6. Bake at 350 degrees F for 20-25 minutes.

7. Cool before serving

Crispy Liver Morsels

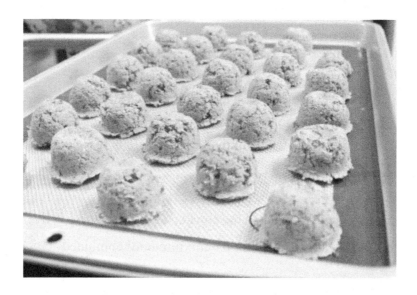

In small amounts, liver is good for cats, and these treats are perfect as part of a healthy diet.

Yield: 12

Total Time: 15mins

Ingredients:

- ½ cup cooked chicken livers (well done)
- ¼ cup water
- 1¼ cups whole wheat flour
- 1 tbsp. soft margarine
- ¼ cup cooked carrot (mashed)

Directions:

1. Preheat the main oven to 325 degrees F.

2. Add the well-done chicken livers in a food blender along with the water.

3. In a mixing bowl, combine the wheat flour along with the margarine. Add the liver mixture to the carrots and using your hands, knead the dough mixture into a ball.

4. Roll the dough out to around ¼" thick and cut into 1" pieces.

5. Arrange the cookies on a lightly greased cookie tray and take in the oven for 10 minutes.

Crunchy Cat Cookies

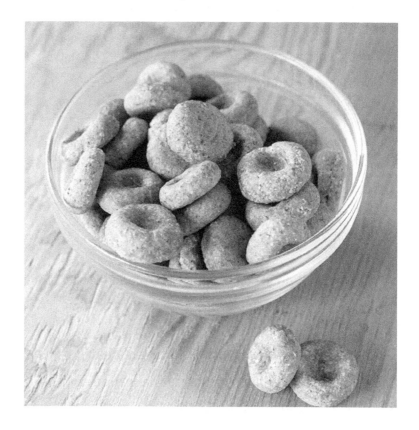

A tempting, tasty treat for your cat companion who will love these sardine infused cookies.

Yield: 14-16 cookies

Total Time: 25mins

Ingredients:

- Non- stick cooking spray
- 1 tin (7 ounces) sardines in oil (mashed)
- ¼ dry non-fat milk
- ½ cup wheat germ

Ingredients:

1. Preheat the main oven to 350 degrees F. Lightly grease a baking sheet with nonstick cooking spray.

2. In a mixing bowl combine the mashed sardines along with the dry nonfat milk and wheat germ.

3. Using a teaspoon, roll out small servings of the mixture into small, grape-sized balls.

4. Arrange each ball onto the baking sheet and using the back of a fork, flatten each ball.

5. Transfer to the oven for between 15-20 minutes, or until the cookies are golden brown.

6. Allow the cookies to cool before giving them to your cat.

7. Store the cookies in an air-tight, lidded container.

Feline Fish Balls

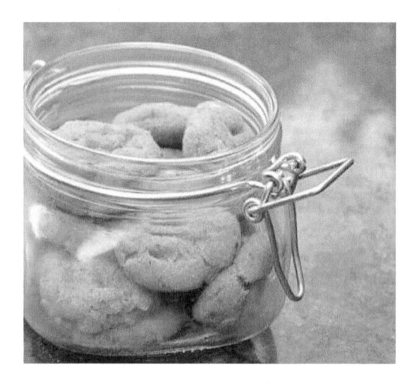

Little balls of fish that easy to make and packed full with all your cat's favorite fishy flavors.

Yield: 16 balls

Total Time: 30mins

Ingredients:

- 2 baby carrots (scrubbed, chopped)
- 1 (15 ounce) tinned tuna in oil
- 2 ounces cooked herring
- 2 tbsp. bread crumbs
- 2 tbsp. cheese (grated)
- 2 tsp Brewer's yeast*
- ¼ tsp catnip (finely chopped)
- 1 medium egg (well beaten)
- 2 tbsp. tomato paste

Directions:

1. Preheat the main oven to 350 degrees F. Lightly grease a baking sheet or tray.

2. In a medium saucepan cook the carrots in boiling water until they are tender. Remove them from the pan and drain.

3. In a large mixing bowl, mash the carrots and add the tuna and herring along with the bread crumbs, grated cheese, brewer's yeast, chopped catnip, beaten egg and tomato paste. Mix until the mixture is silky smooth and the consistency of a thick paste.

4. Roll the mixture into small, evenly sized balls and arrange on the greased baking sheet.

5. Bake them in the preheated oven for 15-20 minutes, or until they are firm and golden-brown

6. Completely cool before serving.

*Ensure that the Brewer's yeast does not contain onion or garlic.

Feline Turkey Loaf

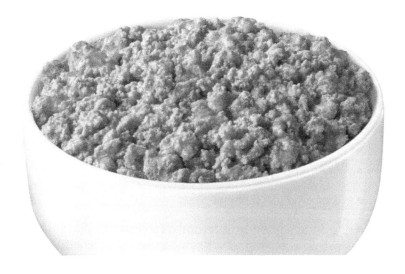

A fabulous Thanksgiving and Christmas meal for your favorite feline and what's more you can freeze this recipe for up to eight weeks.

Yield: 8-10 servings

Total Time: 1hour 40mins

Ingredients:

- Cooking spray
- 1 (7 ounce) can turkey meat (save liquid from can)
- ½ cup mashed sweet potatoes (mashed)
- 2 tbsp. julienne carrots (cooked)
- ½ cup milk (powdered non-fat dry milk mixed with water)
- ¼ cup butter
- 3 egg yolks (beaten)
- 2-3 cups plain breadcrumbs (reserve 1 tablespoon of bread crumbs for top)
- 3 egg whites (exceptionally well beaten)
- 1 tsp anchovy paste mixed with 1 tablespoon ketchup
- 1 tsp dried fish flakes

Directions

1. Pre-heat the main oven to 350 degrees F.

2. Lightly mist a loaf pan with cooking spray.

3. Drain the canned turkey meat and set the liquid to one side and transfer to a food blender.

4. Add the sweet potatoes and cooked carrots to the turkey and blitz until combined.

5. In a saucepan heat the milk along with the butter, and gently simmer until just boiling. Remove the pan from heat and put to one side for 5 minutes.

6. In a separate mixing bowl, whip the egg yolks

7. Add the liquid set aside earlier from the canned turkey to the egg yolk mix, and blend until silky smooth.

8. Add the ingredients from the blender to the egg yolks and mix well to combine.

9. Add the milk-butter mixture to the egg yolks and blend to incorporate.

10. Add the bread crumbs, saving 1 tablespoon for the top, and mix well.

11. Next, fold in the egg whites and pour them into a greased loaf pan.

12. Spread the anchovy paste mixture across the top of the whole loaf.

13. Sprinkle dried fish flakes and the reserved bread crumbs over the top.

14. Bake in the oven for at least 1½ hours until sufficiently cooked. A cocktail inserted in the middle of the loaf comes out clean.

15. Remove from the oven, and allow to cool. Once cool, slice into sections approximately ¼" thick and serve.

Fruit for Felines

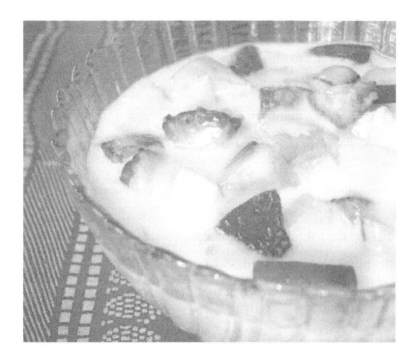

If you want to replace high-calorie cat treats with fresh produce then remember that a little fresh fruit now and again is perfectly acceptable.

Yield: 6 cups

Total Time: 3mins

Ingredients:

- 2 cups fresh cantaloupe (cut into small pieces)
- 3 cups fresh watermelon (cut into small pieces)
- 1 cup fresh blueberries
- Splash unsweetened soy milk
- Nutritional yeast (to garnish)

Directions:

1. Add the cantaloupe and watermelon to a bowl. Next, add the blueberries and a splash of milk. Sprinkle the nutritional yeast over the top. Serve at room temperature.

Kitty Bites

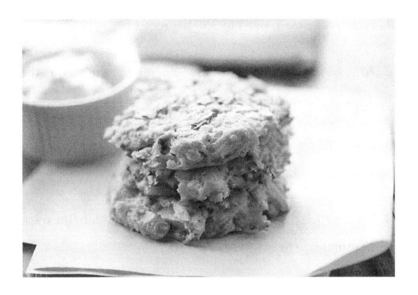

Your cat will find these bites the purrfect snack.

Yield: 12 bites

Total Time: 12mins

Ingredients:

- 1 (5 ounce) can of tuna
- ½ cup white cornmeal
- ½ cup flour
- ½ cup water

Directions:

1. Preheat the main oven to 350 degrees F.

2. In a bowl, combine all 4 ingredients together until the mixture forms a ball.

3. Break off tiny pieces of the mixture and roll out into even bite size balls and place on a baking sheet.

4. Flatten each ball using your finger and transfer to the oven for 5 minutes.

5. Flip the bites over and bake for a further 4-5 minutes.

6. Allow to cool before serving.

Kitty Breakfast

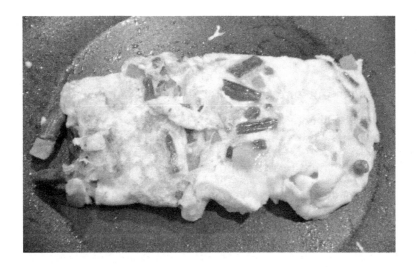

When you sit down to your pancakes and syrup why not spoil kitty with this protein-rich breakfast.

Yield: 2-3 servings

Total Time: 10mins

Ingredients:

- 1 tbsp. non-fat dry milk
- Water
- 3 medium eggs
- 3 tbsp. cottage cheese
- 2 tbsp. grated veggies (grated)

Directions:

1. Combine the milk powder along with a drop of water. Add the eggs and beat well to incorporate.

2. Add the mixture to a nonstick frying pan and over medium to low heat, cook until done.

3. Flip the mixture over, and evenly spoon the cottage cheese and grated vegetables over half of the cooked mixture.

4. Fold over, as you would an omelet and when cool, cut into bite-sized pieces.

Kitty Bruschetta

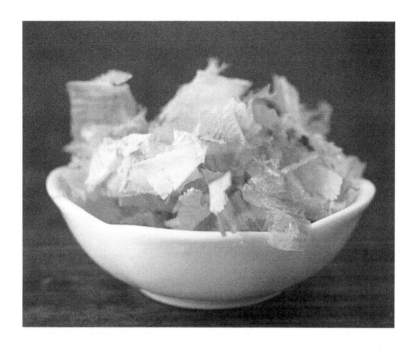

A three ingredient, quick and easy treat that is sure to get your cat purring.

Yield: 2 servings

Total Time: 10mins

Ingredients:

- 1 slice of bread
- Fresh fish oil

- Dried fish flakes

Directions:

1. Very lightly toast one slice of bread and cut into 1" cubes.

2. Brush the tops of each cube with fish oil and scatter with dried fish flakes.

3. Bake in the oven at 350 degrees F, or until the cubes are golden.

4. Allow the kitty bruschetta to cool a little before servings.

Kitty's Favorite Turkey Balls

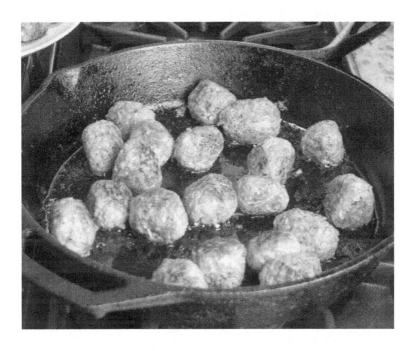

Tasty meatballs that your cat won't be able to resist.

Yield: 12-14 small meatballs

Total Time: 25mins

Ingredients:

- ½ pound ground turkey
- ½ cup carrots (grated)
- ¼ cup cottage cheese

- ½ cup crackers (finely crushed)
- ¼ cup powdered milk
- 1 medium egg
- 1 tbsp. Brewer's yeast*
- ½ tsp salt

Directions:

1. Preheat the main oven to 350 degrees F.

2. Using clean hands combine all the ingredients together in a large mixing bowl.

3. Mold the mixture into nuggets, the size of golf balls, and place them in a nonstick baking pan.

4. Transfer the pan to the oven for 18-20 minutes, or until they are golden brown and have an internal temperature of around 160 degrees F.

5. Allow the turkey balls to cool before serving.

*Ensure that the Brewer's yeast does not contain onion or garlic.

Liver Cake

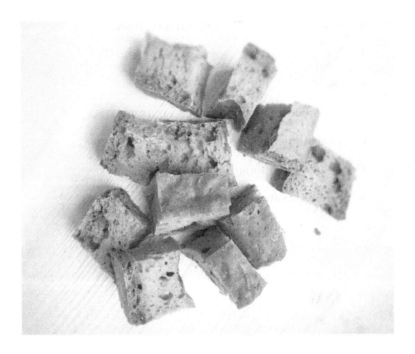

A wheat-free treat or meal topping that is totally nutritious.

Yield: 10-12 servings

Total Time: 1hour

Ingredients:

- ½ lb. fresh raw organic chicken liver
- 2 free-range eggs (beaten)
- 4 tbsp. vegetable oil
- 3 tbsp. unsweetened canned pumpkin
- 1 cups instant oats
- 2 tbsp. nutritional yeast (optional)
- Filtered water (for the batter)

Directions:

1. Preheat the main oven to 350 degrees F.

2. In a food blender, process the chicken liver, until a puree is formed; this will take 2-3 minutes.

3. Add the beaten eggs to a bowl and add the vegetable oil. Next, add the pureed liver to the bowl.

4. Add the dry ingredients a little at a time, while stirring, until combined. Gradually add the water until a batter-like consistency is achieved.

5. Pour the batter into a cake tin and bake in the preheated oven for 45-50 minutes, or until the cake is firm.

6. Allow the cake to cook in the tin, and when it is cool enough to handle, gently place it on a baking rack and transfer it to the refrigerator until cool.

7. Using a sharp knife slice and dice the cake into bite-size pieces.

Mackerel for Moggies!

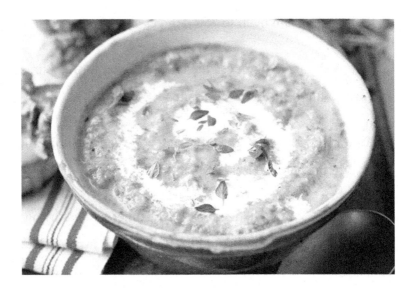

This recipe is a good one for the newbie, homemade cat recipe cook.

Yield: 1-2 servings

Total Time: 5mins

Ingredients:

- 1 cup canned mackerel
- 1 tbsp. sunflower seed oil
- 1 tbsp. cooked brown rice
- 1-2 tbsp. of chicken broth

Directions:

1. Add the 4 ingredients to a food blender and pulse until incorporated.

2. Serve immediately.

Meat and Oats Cat Food

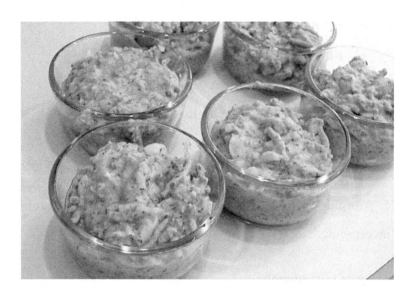

Cats can benefit from a small portion of oatmeal. Remember, though your cat needs to have plenty of animal protein so this recipe is purrrfect.

Yield: 2-3 servings

Total Time: 20mins

Ingredients:

- 1 cup rolled oats
- 3 cups water
- 1 hard-boiled egg (cold)
- 2 tbsp. vegetable oil
- 1 pound minced beef
- 1 tbsp. spinach (finely chopped)

Directions:

1. In a saucepan, boil the oats in cold water until they absorb the water and become soft.

2. Using a fork, mash the hard-boiled egg into the cooked oats.

3. In a frying pan, add the vegetable oil along with the minced beef and cook thoroughly.

4. Add the cooked beef to the oat-egg mixture and stir in the spinach.

5. Stir well to fully incorporate.

6. Allow to cool before serving.

Oatmeal Sardine Treats

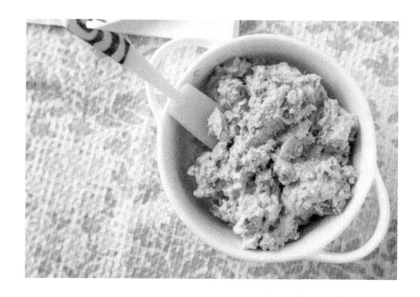

Oatmeal is fine for cats as long as it doesn't contain milk, so this recipe is ideal.

Yield: 4-6 treats

Total Time: 5mins

Ingredients:

- 1 can sardines in oil
- 2 tbsp. carrot (grated)
- ⅓ cup oatmeal (cooked)

Directions:

1. Combine all 3 ingredients in a mixing bowl and mash to incorporate.

Peanut Butter Cat Treats

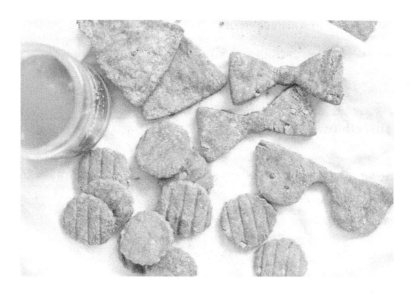

Raw peanut butter can cause your cat to choke but these tempting treats are baked in the oven and so are easy for your cat to nibble.

Yield: 18-20 treats

Total Time: 20mins

Ingredients:

- ½ cup buckwheat flour
- ½ cup quinoa flour
- ¼ tsp baking soda
- ½ cup smooth, organic peanut butter
- ½ cup unsweetened applesauce

Directions:

1. Preheat the main oven to 350 degrees F.

2. In a bowl, stir the flours into the baking soda and set to one side.

3. In a mixing bowl, combine the peanut butter along with the applesauce until silky smooth. Scrape it into the flour mixture and stir until it is hard to stir. Finally, incorporating the flour by kneading it into the dough.

4. Roll the dough out to ¼ "thickness and transfer it to an ungreased cookie tray or sheet.

5. Bake in the preheated oven for 10 minutes.

6. Transfer it to a chopping board and cut into bite-sized cat treats. Arrange the cut treats on the cookie sheet and bake for a couple more minutes.

7. Allow to cool before serving.

8. Store for up to 14 days in an airtight container in the refrigerator.

Purrfect Pumpkin Pie Treats

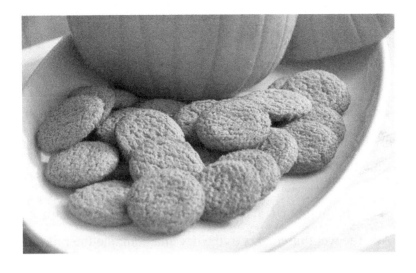

Your cat can join in the fall festivities with this pumpkin inspired treat recipe.

Yield: 30-40 treats

Total Time: 20mins

Ingredients:

- 1 cup canned pumpkin
- ½ cup unsweetened plain applesauce
- 1 cup carrots (grated)
- 2 cups brown rice flour
- ½ cup uncooked oatmeal

- ¼ cup brown rice flour (for rolling)

Directions:

1. Preheat the main oven to 350 degrees.

2. In a food blender or processor blend the canned pumpkin, along with the applesauce and grated carrots until silky smooth.

3. In a mixing bowl, add the flour together with the oatmeal. Add the wet ingredients to the dry and combine the mixture by hand until a dough forms.

4. On a clean work surface, dusted with flour, roll the dough out to around ¼" thick. Using a cookie cutter form shapes.

5. Arrange the cookies on a lightly greased cookie sheet and bake in the oven for 7 minutes.

6. Flipping the treats over, bake for an additional 5-6 minutes.

7. Remove the treats from the oven and allow to cool.

8. Store in the refrigerator for up to 8 weeks in an airtight container.

Rabbit Stew

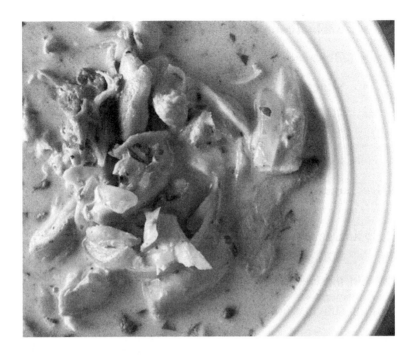

This recipe is one that you can share with your feline friend as it's a tasty meal for humans, too.

Yield: 6-8 servings

Total Time: 2hours

Ingredients:

- Rabbit (boned, cut into small pieces)
- Olive oil
- Vegetable stock (unsalted)
- Sweet potato, carrot, celery, turnip, and peas
- Springs of parsley, rosemary, marjoram, and thyme

Directions:

1. In a large frying pan sauté the pieces of rabbit in olive oil.

2. Add the vegetable stock and bring to a swift boil. When boiling, cover with a lid and cook over medium-low heat until cooked through.

3. Next, add the vegetables and herbs, cook for a further 40-45 minutes.

4. Allow the stew to cool before serving to your cat.

Salad Bowl

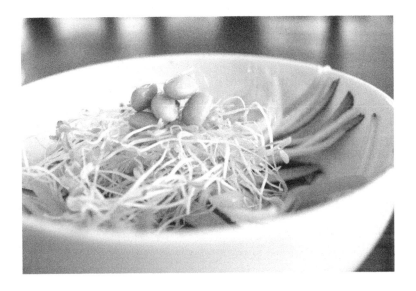

Add some greens to a salad for your cat to enjoy. Alfalfa greens provide fiber, protein and vitamin K and will satisfy kitty's need for something green.

Yield: 1-2 servings

Total Time: 5mins

Ingredients:

- ½ cup alfalfa sprouts (finely chopped)
- ¼ cup zucchini (grated)
- 2 tbsp. chicken stock
- ⅛ tsp catnip (minced, optional)

Directions:

1. In a mixing bowl, toss the alfalfa sprouts with the zucchini and chicken stock.

2. Scatter over the catnip (if required) and serve.

3. The salad can be refrigerated in an airtight, container for up to 48 hours.

Salmon Delight

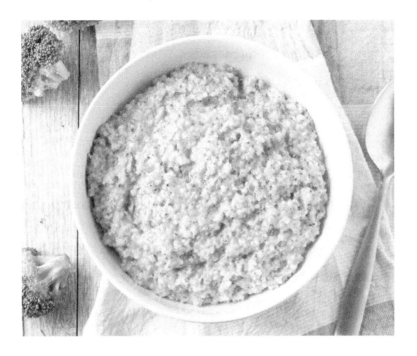

All cats love fish but did you know that they should only be fed tuna and salmon as an occasional treat.

Yield: 1-2 servings

Total Time: 5mins

Ingredients:

- 1 (2½ ounce) can salmon
- 1 tbsp. broccoli (cooked, mashed)
- ¼ cup whole wheat bread crumbs
- 1 tsp Brewer's yeast*

Directions:

1. Combine all 4 ingredients in a mixing bowl, mash together and serve.

*Check that the Brewer's yeast does not contain garlic or onions.

Sardine Cookies

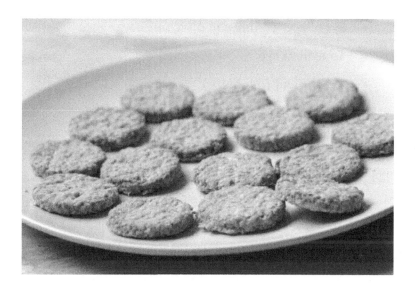

With just three simple ingredients you can bake up a batch of simple sardine cookies.

Yield: 12-14 cookies

Total Time: 20mins

Ingredients:

- 3¾ ounces sardines in olive oil
- 1 medium egg
- ½ cup flour (of choice)

Directions:

1. Preheat the main oven to 350 degrees F.

2. First, puree the sardines along with their oil and mix in the egg,

3. Add the flour, a little at a time, until the mixture is a cookie dough consistency.

4. Take a teaspoon of the dough and roll the mixture into a ball.

5. Transfer the balls to an ungreased cookie tray and gently flatten each ball, using the back of a fork.

6. Place in the oven for between 12-15 minutes, or until the cookies are gently browned.

7. Allow the cookies to cool on a wire baking rack and store in an airtight, lidded container for up to 7 days.

Sardine Sea Balls Cat Treats

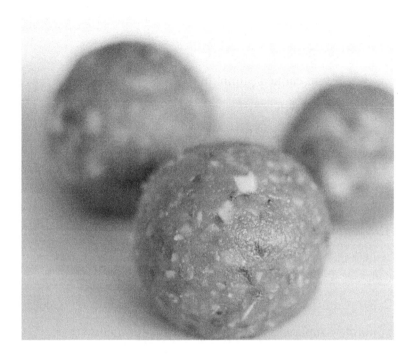

Pumpkin is great for your furry friend's digestion and can, in fact, help to prevent hairballs.

Yield: 12 treats

Total Time: 10mins

Ingredients:

- 1 cup boneless, skinless low-sodium canned sardines (drained)
- ½ cup canned pumpkin
- 1 tbsp. fish oil
- 1 tbsp. kelp

Directions:

1. Mix all 4 ingredients together in a mixing bowl. Using your hands, roll the mixture into small treat size balls.

2. Store in the refrigerator for up to 3 days, in a re-sealable container, separating each layer with parchment paper.

Savory Cheesy Treats

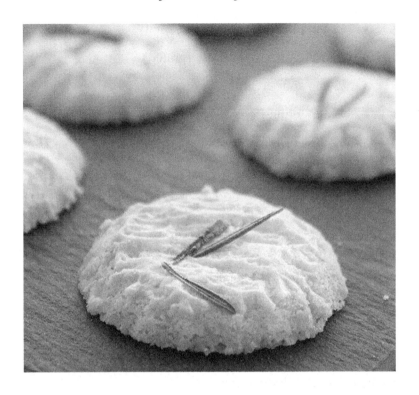

Small amounts of cheese aren't harmful to your cat but remember treats should never represent more than 10% of your pet's daily calorie intake.

Yield: 24

Total Time: 35mins

Ingredients:

- ¾ cup cheddar cheese (shredded)
- 5 tbsp. Parmesan cheese (grated)
- ¼ cup sour cream
- ¾ cup white flour
- ¼ cup cornmeal

Directions:

1. Preheat the main oven to 350 degrees F.

2. In a bowl combine the cheddar cheese, Parmesan cheese, and sour cream.

3. Add the flour and cornmeal and add a little water to achieve a dough-like mixture.

4. Using your hands, knead the dough into a ball and roll out to ¼".

5. Cut the dough into 1" sized pieces and transfer to a lightly greased cookie tray or sheet and bake for 25 minutes.

6. Allow to cool before serving.

Shrimp and Carrots

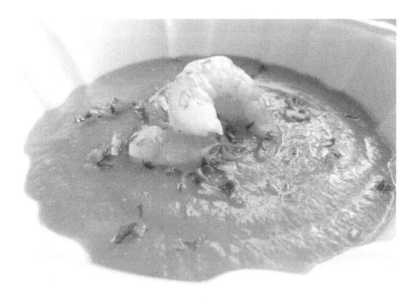

Cats love shrimp but did you know they like carrots too? Cooked carrots are way better than raw because they don't present a choking hazard.

Yield: 2 servings

Total Time: 30mins

Ingredients:

- 4 large shrimp (uncooked)
- 2 medium carrots (scrubbed, chopped)

Directions:

1. First, prepare the shrimps by cutting off their tails and removing their outside layers.

2. In a nonstick frying pan and on low heat, sauté the shrimps until cooked through.

3. In a saucepan, filled with boiling water, boil the carrots for 10-15 minutes. Allow the carrots to cool and transfer to a food blender and process until silky smooth; this will only take a few seconds.

4. As soon as the shrimps have cooled, cut them into small bite-size pieces.

5. Combine the carrots with the shrimps and serve.

Simple Ground Beef

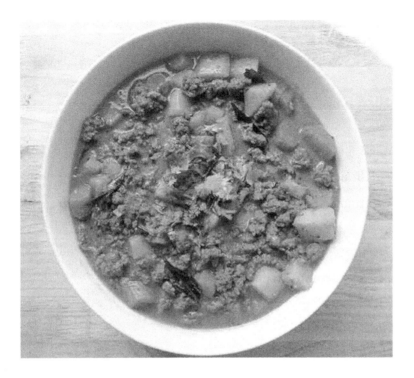

Lots of protein in this simple cat food recipe which is great for cats as they metabolize amino acids very quickly and they need protein for their bodies to function effectively.

Yield: 3-4 servings

Total Time: 30mins

Ingredients:

- ¼ pound ground beef
- Water

Directions:

1. In a saucepan over high heat cook the ground beef in a small amount of water, that is just enough to help it cook. Continue cooking until there is no pink meat left.

2. Allow to cool before transferring to a food blender and processing until smooth.

Stool Softener Treat

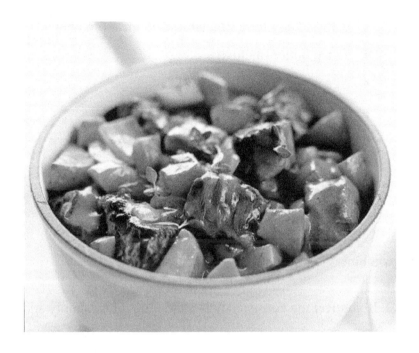

If your cat is having a problem passing a stool, wait 24 hours and then give them this treat.

Yield: 1 serving

Total Time: 10mins

Ingredients:

- 1 tbsp. baby food vegetables and meat (no onions!)
- ½ tsp butter (melted)
- ⅛ tsp ground psyllium husks
- ⅛ tsp powdered bran
- 2 tbsp. cold water

Directions:

1. Combine all 5 ingredients in a small bowl and mix to combine.

2. If you feel the consistency is a little too thick, simply add a drop more water.

Surf and Turf

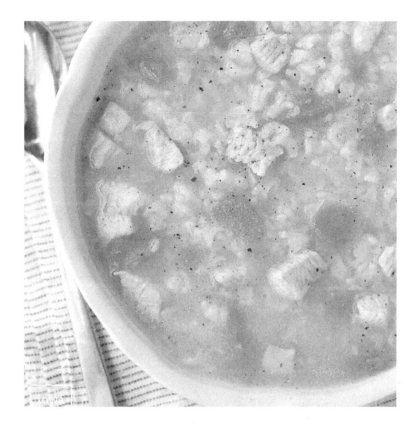

Why not indulge your furry friend once in a while and whip up this animal-friendly surf and turf.

Yield: 1-2 servings

Total Time: 5mins

Ingredients:

- ½ cup white chicken meat (cooked)
- 1 (5 ounces) can tuna in sunflower oil
- 1 tbsp. carrot cooked (mashed)
- 2 tbsp. brown rice

Directions:

1. Combine all 4 ingredients in a food blender or processor and blitz until combined.

2. Store in the fridge for up to 72 hours.

Thanksgiving Turkey Nibblers

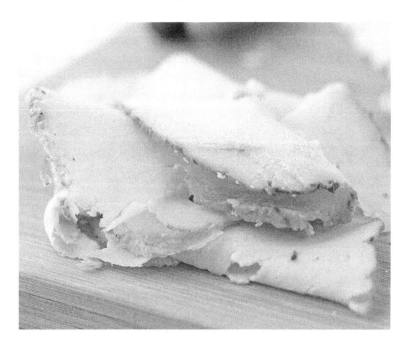

Your cat will love these turkey strips, and it's a great way to use up any Thanksgiving leftovers.

Yield: 12

Total Time: 11hours 7mins

Ingredients:

- Cooking spray
- 12 strips dark turkey meat (thinly sliced, bone-free)

Directions:

1. Preheat the oven to 300 degrees F. Lightly spray a cookie tray or sheet with nonstick cooking spray.

2. Remove any skin or fat from the meat and using a sharp knife, cut the turkey into 1" slices.

3. Arrange the strips on the cookie tray and bake for 2½ -3 hours. While they are baking, make sure that they don't burn by checking them constantly.

4. Turn the oven off but leave the turkey strips in the oven for between 6-8 hours until totally cool.

The Cat's Meow Meal

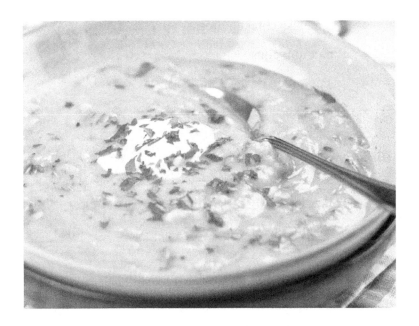

This recipe is the cat's whiskers! Your cat will love the combination of chicken, and green beans. Don't forget though to make sure that the chicken is bone free.

Yield: 2-3 servings

Total Time: 1hour

Ingredients:

- 1 boneless chicken breast
- 2 medium eggs
- ½ cup green beans (chopped)
- ½ tsp fish sauce

Directions:

1. Cook the chicken breast until its juices run clear. Shred the chicken into bite-size pieces.

2. Add the cooked chicken along with the eggs in a microwave safe bowl and cook on full power for 2-3 minutes, or until the eggs are cooked.

3. Add the beans along with the fish sauce.

4. Set to one side to cool.

The Klassic Kat Recipe

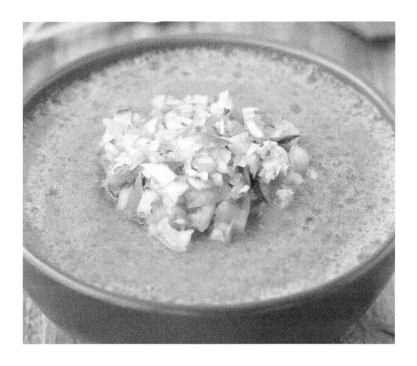

A simple recipe that is packed full of goodness to help keep your furry friend happy and healthy.

Yield: 1-2 servings

Total Time: 10mins

Ingredients:

- 2 tbsp. mixed orange and green veggies (carrots, zucchini, sweet potato, etc.)
- ½ cup raw meat (cut into chunks)
- ¾ tsp edible human bone meal
- 1 raw egg yolk

Directions:

1. In a food blender finely grind the vegetables.

2. In a bowl combine the remaining ingredients to make a chili-like consistency. Add a drop of cold water if you feel the mixture is too dry.

3. Gently warm the food by setting your cat's food bowl in warm water.

Trout Dinner

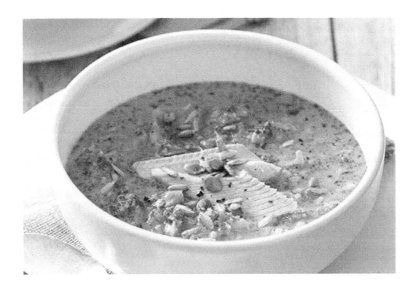

Spoil your cat with this gourmet trout dinner.

Yield: 1¼ cups

Total Time: 5mins

Ingredients:

- 1 cup cooked trout
- 1 egg yolk (cooked)
- 1 tbsp. steamed broccoli (chopped small)
- 2 tbsp. sunflower oil

Directions:

1. Combine all 4 ingredients in a food blender or processor and blitz until combined.

2. Store in the fridge for up to 72 hours.

Tuna Pumpkin Biscotti Treats

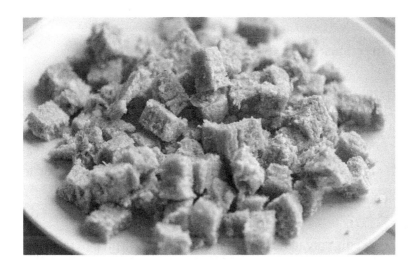

Spelt flour is very easy on your cat's digestive system. These treats are particularly good because you can bake up a batch and store them for up to 8 weeks in the refrigerator.

Yield: 18-20 treats

Total Time: 1hour 30mins

Ingredients:

- 1 cup whole-spelt flour
- 1 can low-sodium tuna in water (do not drain)
- 1 medium egg
- 2 tbsp. extra-virgin light olive oil

- Pinch salt
- ½ cup canned pumpkin

Directions:

1. Preheat the main oven to 350 degrees F. Line a cookie tray or sheet with parchment paper.

2. In a mixing bowl combine all the ingredients and stir to incorporate.

3. Evenly spread the dough mixture onto the prepared cookie tray to around 1/8" thickness.

4. Transfer to the oven and bake for 20 minutes. Remove from the oven and all to cool for 4-5 minutes.

5. Flip the sheet of treats, peel off the parchment paper and continue baking for 8 minutes.

6. Turn off the oven and allow the tray of treats to rest for 60 minutes, or until crisp.

7. Remove the treats and allow to cool on a baking rake before cutting into strips of approximately 2x1" strips.

8. Store in the fridge or freeze.

Tuna Tiddlebits

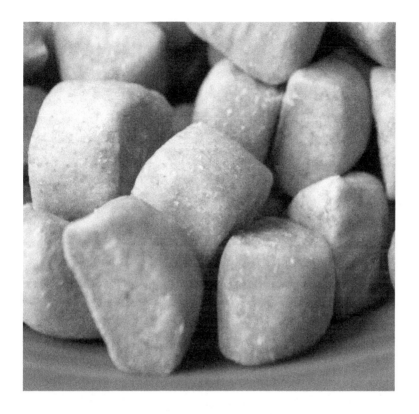

Tasty little tuna fish cookies for Tiddles. Too much canned fish isn't good for your cat but served as a treat it's fine.

Yield: 12

Total Time: 25mins

Ingredients:

- 1(6 ounce) can of tuna
- ¼ cup tuna fish water drained from tuna
- 3 tbsp. cooked egg white (chopped)
- ¼ cup cornmeal
- ½ cup whole wheat flour

Directions:

1. Preheat the main oven to 350 degrees F.

2. In a mixing bowl combine the tuna, tuna water and egg white and stir.

3. Add the cornmeal and whole wheat flour and blend until dough is formed.

4. Using your hand knead the mixture into a ball and roll out to around ¼" thick.

5. Cut the dough into 1" sized piece and bake in the oven for 20 minutes.

Author's Afterthoughts

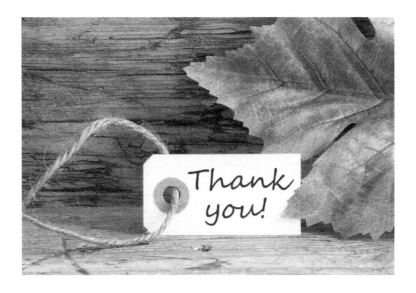

Thanks ever so much to each of my cherished readers for investing the time to read this book!

I know you could have picked from many other books but you chose this one. So, a big thanks for downloading this book and reading all the way to the end.

If you enjoyed this book or received value from it, I'd like to ask you for a favor. Please take a few minutes to post an honest and heartfelt review on Amazon.com. Your support does make a difference and helps to benefit other people.

Thanks!

Daniel Humphreys

About the Author

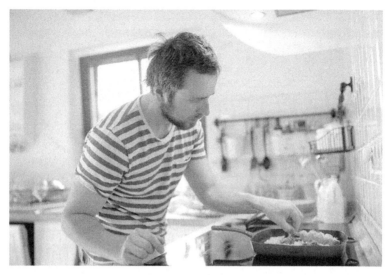

Daniel Humphreys

Many people will ask me if I am German or Norman, and my answer is that I am 100% unique! Joking aside, I owe my cooking influence mainly to my mother who was British! I can certainly make a mean Sheppard's pie, but when it comes to preparing Bratwurst sausages and drinking beer with friends, I am also all in!

I am taking you on this culinary journey with me and hope you can appreciate my diversified background. In my 15 years career as a chef, I never had a dish returned to me by one of clients, so that should say something about me! Actually, I will take that back. My worst critic is my four years old son, who refuses to taste anything that is green color. That shall pass, I am sure.

My hope is to help my children discover the joy of cooking and sharing their creations with their loved ones, like I did all my life. When you develop a passion for cooking and my suspicious is that you have one as well, it usually sticks for life. The best advice I can give anyone as a professional chef is invest. Invest your time, your heart in each meal you are creating. Invest also a little money in good cooking hardware and quality ingredients. But most of all enjoy every meal you prepare with YOUR friends and family!

Made in the USA
Las Vegas, NV
13 February 2021